CONTENTS

Words appearing in the text in bold, **like this**, are explained in the Glossary.

THE HORMONAL SYSTEM

The human body has hundreds of major parts, like the stomach, liver, **kidneys**, brain, bones, muscles and heart. Each of these carries out important tasks. However, all these parts must work together, in a controlled and coordinated way, so the body can function as a whole and stay healthy.

Two systems in the body carry out control and coordination. They are the **nervous system** and the **endocrine system**. The endocrine system works using substances called hormones. These are natural chemicals made by body parts known as endocrine **glands**.

Although they are produced in glands, the effects of hormones are felt all over the body. The hormonal system has three main tasks:
- to control the level of many substances, and the speed of many chemical processes, so that conditions inside the body remain stable. For example, hormones will ensure that, when you exercise your body, enough energy is released for your body to cope with the extra activity.
- to help the body react to **stressful** conditions, like an exam or an interview
- to regulate the body's growth and development from baby to adult, and throughout life.

The needs of your body change depending on whether you are sleeping, studying or exercising. Hormones are concerned with managing your body's internal environment so that these needs are met. This process is called homeostasis.

Hormone-making glands

There are about twelve major endocrine glands. Another ten or so organs, like the stomach and heart, have other main tasks to do, but they also make some hormones. There are more than 100 different hormones. Many of their names end with 'in' or 'ine', like **insulin** and **adrenaline**.

Hormones and their targets

Hormones are released into the blood, and as the blood circulates around the body they are carried to all parts of the body. However, each hormone only affects certain parts of the body, known as its targets. Some hormones have just one target, such as gastrin, which makes the stomach produce more digestive juices. Other hormones affect several targets. A few hormones, such as growth hormone and thyroxine, affect most parts of the body.

Hormones

Injury, Illness and Health

Steve Parker

www.heinemann.co.uk/library
Visit our website to find out more information about **Heinemann Library** books.

To order:
☎ Phone 44 (0) 1865 888066
▤ Send a fax to 44 (0) 1865 314091
▯ Visit the Heinemann Bookshop at www.heinemann.co.uk/library to browse our
catalogue and order online.

First published in Great Britain by Heinemann
Library, Halley Court, Jordan Hill, Oxford
OX2 8EJ, part of Harcourt Education.

Heinemann is a registered trademark of Harcourt
Education Ltd.

Editorial: Nick Hunter and Catherine Clarke
Design: Jo Hinton-Malivoire and
Tinstar Design Limited (www.tinstar.co.uk)
Illustrations: Art Construction except for p.5 by
Ken Vail Graphic Design
Picture Research: Maria Joannou and
Su Alexander
Production: Viv Hichens

Originated by Ambassador Litho Ltd
Printed in Hong Kong, China by
Wing King Tong Company Limited

ISBN 0 431 15718 9 (hardback)
07 06 05 04 03
10 9 8 7 6 5 4 3 2 1

ISBN 0 431 15725 1 (paperback)
08 07 06 05 04 03
10 9 8 7 6 5 4 3 2 1

British Library Cataloguing in Publication Data
Parker, Steve
Hormones. – (Body Focus)
612. 4' 05
A full catalogue record for this book is available
from the British Library.

Acknowledgements
The publishers would like to thank the following
for permission to reproduce photographs:

Corbis pp. 15 (Bill Varie), 43 (Anthony Redpath);
Corbis Bettmann p. 41, Corbis Stockmarket pp.
10 (George Schiavone), 16 (Tim Pannell), 29 (Jim
Cummins), 38 (Darama); Getty Images pp.11, 21,
31, 32, 36; Science Photo Library pp. 6 (Astrid &
Hans-Frieder Michler), 7 (Professor K Seddon &
Dr T. Evans, Queens University, Belfast), 9
(Susumu Nishinaga), 12 (Scott Camazine), 14
(Simon Fraser), 18 (Mehau Kulyk), 20 (Alfred
Pasieka), 23 (Damien Lovegrove), 24 (John Paul
Kay, Peter Arnold Inc.), 25 (Richard Menga,
Fundamental Photos), 26 (CNRI), 30 (Russell D.
Curtis), 33 (GJLP), 34 (Biophoto Associates), 37
(Alfred Pasieka), 40 (Josh Sher), 42 (Pascal
Goetgheluck).

Cover photograph of a scan of a healthy thyroid
gland reproduced with permission of Science
Photo Library.

The publishers would like to thank David
Wright for his assistance with the preparation
of this book.

Every effort has been made to contact copyright
holders of any material reproduced in this book.
Any omissions will be rectified in subsequent
printings if notice is given to the publishers.

Hormones and well-being

Hormones and their glands cannot be 'exercised' like muscles can. So hormones may not seem important to fitness and well-being, but they are vital. In particular, they are greatly affected by aspects of lifestyle, such as physical activity, diet, substance abuse, emotions, stress and worry. Following a healthy lifestyle can prevent many hormonal problems.

This diagram shows the body's main hormonal glands. Both the male and female glands are shown here, although they would not normally be found in the same body.

Each hormone is made and released by an endocrine gland and in many cases, this gland is a target for other hormones. The result is that various hormones control each other, in a complex and interrelated way. Also, hormones work alongside the nervous system, and the two systems interact in many ways. They affect each other, and the same targets. The chief link between the two systems is an endocrine gland called the **pituitary**, at the base of the brain.

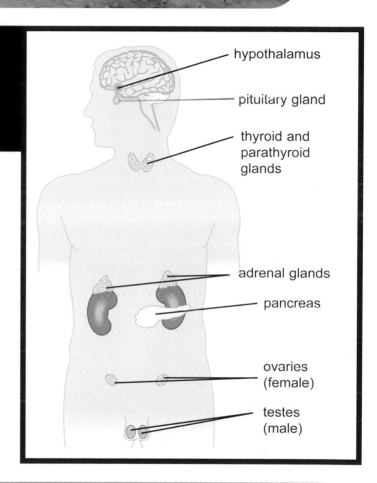

- hypothalamus
- pituitary gland
- thyroid and parathyroid glands
- adrenal glands
- pancreas
- ovaries (female)
- testes (male)

Glands

A gland makes a product, usually a fluid, for use by the body or for removal. Exocrine glands, like tiny sweat glands in the skin, release their products along tubes or ducts.

Endocrine glands, which make hormones, pass their products directly into the blood flowing through them. They are sometimes called ductless glands. The term 'gland' is sometimes used for lymph nodes, which are parts of the body's disease-fighting **immune system**. They swell as the body battles against germs during an infection.

WHAT IS A HORMONE?

Hormones are sometimes called 'chemical messengers'. They are chemicals that carry a particular message or instruction. Because hormones travel in the bloodstream, they come into contact with all parts of the body. However, only certain parts, their targets, respond to the messages.

Usually, a hormone's message makes its target work faster, or make more of its product, or release its contents. The greater the amount, or concentration, of the hormone in the blood, then the greater its effect.

Structure of hormones

Like many other chemicals, hormones consist of identical units called **molecules**. Compared to other molecules in the body, like the **DNA** of the genetic material, or **proteins** that build muscles and bones, hormones are very tiny. They are too small to see, even with the most powerful microscopes.

There are three main chemical groups of hormones:
- **amines**
- **peptides**
- **steroids**.

The differences between them are important because the groups work in different ways, and this affects how extra hormones may be given to treat people with hormonal problems.

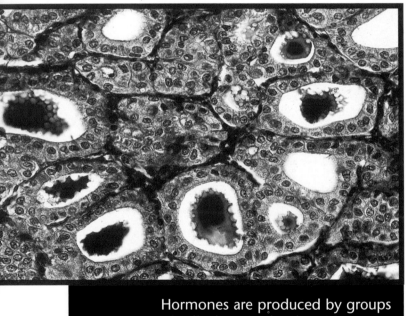

Hormones are produced by groups of cells, here in the thyroid.

Substance abuse

The hormonal system is a chemical system. It is especially at risk from unusual or strange chemicals put into the body, such as drugs. Sometimes the damage caused by a drug shows few signs, until it is well advanced. It may then be too late to treat. This is one reason why it is so important to avoid substance abuse.

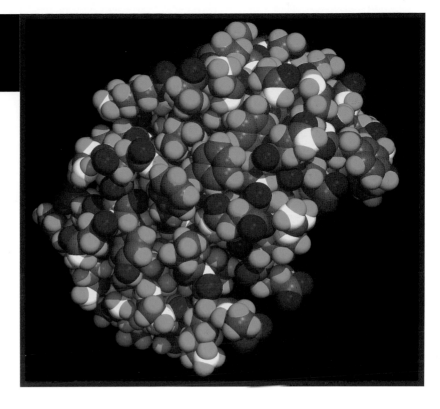

Many atoms join to make a molecule of insulin.

How hormones work

The whole body is made of billions and billions of microscopic parts known as cells. A cell is like a bag, or container of substances enclosed in a 'skin' – the cell **membrane**. On the cell membrane are special sites known as **receptors**. A typical body cell has millions of receptors, of various kinds, on its cell membrane. The exact kinds of receptors determine which hormones affect that cell – that is, whether the cell is a target for the hormone. A molecule of a certain hormone slots into a receptor of a similar shape, like a key fitting into a lock. When this happens, the hormone 'switches on' production of another substance within the cell, which causes the hormone's effect.

Most amine or peptide hormones work in this way. Steroid hormones, which include the anti-**stress** hormone cortisol, and the hormones involved with the sex organs, have a slightly different action. They also fit into receptors, like keys into locks, but these receptors are inside the cell. The molecules of hormone must first pass through the cell membrane, to gain access to the receptors inside, so they can 'switch on' their target process.

Slow and fast

The hormonal and **nervous systems** work closely together, to regulate and coordinate the body's many parts. There are basic differences however, especially in terms of the speed of action. The hormonal system tends to act slowly, over hours, days, weeks and years, for long-term effects, such as the slow growth of a child into an adult over many years. The nervous system works faster, over seconds and even fractions of a second. For example, the immediate pain you feel when you touch something hot.

HORMONES AND FEEDBACK

Most hormones exert their effect using a system called the feedback loop. Usually, as the level of a hormone rises in the body, its target becomes more active. Sensors in the body detect the amount of hormone and the activity of the target that hormone affects. They 'feedback' this information via a control centre, most often in the brain, to the **endocrine gland** that makes and releases the hormone.

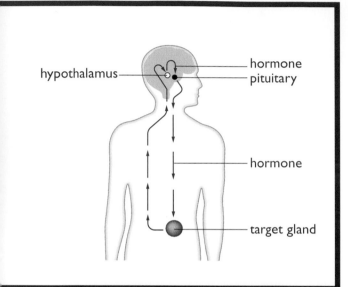

A feedback loop involves the brain, hormone and target gland.

Switching on and off

When the required level of the hormone is reached, or its target is working in the way the body needs, feedback 'switches off' the hormone's release. The level of hormone falls, and its target becomes less active. This happens until a lower limit is reached, which is again detected by the sensors. The system then 'switches on' again, and so on.

In this way the level of the hormone and the activity of its target vary between set limits. The chief aim of the feedback system is to maintain suitable conditions inside the body, so that all parts can work well, despite the body's changing activities and needs throughout the day.

Feedback sensors

For most hormones, the sensors are tiny clusters of cells, often smaller than pinheads. They monitor the concentration of their hormone and/or the product that their target makes, in the blood passing through them. Many of these sensors are in, or near the **hypothalamus**, a part at the base of the brain, or the **pituitary**, which is the small endocrine gland just below it. This is often called the 'master gland' because the pituitary and the hypothalamus work closely together as the dual control centres for much of the body's hormonal activity.

An example of feedback

One example of the feedback system concerns the hormone thyroxine. It is made by the **thyroid**, a gland in the front of the neck. Thyroxine's targets are most cells in the body. It makes them work faster, to carry out their chemical processes at an increased rate, thereby using more oxygen and producing more heat. The general term for the millions of chemical processes constantly occurring in the body is **metabolism**. So thyroxine increases metabolic rate.

Chain reactions

As the level of thyroxine falls, so does metabolic rate. This could make the whole body slow down and become dangerously cold. The level of thyroxine is detected by sensors in the hypothalamus. This releases its own hormone, TRH (thyrotropin-releasing hormone). TRH passes to the pituitary just below it, where it causes release of another hormone, TSH (thyroid-stimulating hormone). TSH travels around the body in the blood. It causes the thyroid to release more thyroxine, which makes the body's metabolic rate increase.

In this feedback loop, one hormone affects another, which then controls another, in a 'chain reaction'. Such multiple control is quite common in the hormonal system.

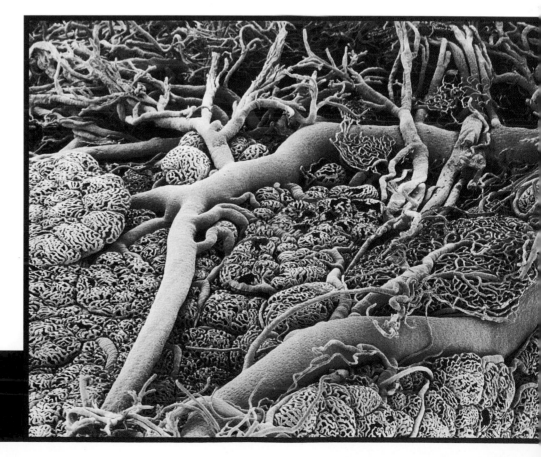

Hormones travel in tiny blood vessels, capillaries, to every body part.

People can improve their health and prevent illness in many ways. Exercise strengthens muscles and joints, and a balanced diet keeps the **digestive system** working well. However, we don't usually think of the hormonal system in this way. It is often seen as a 'fixed' part of the body, which cannot be altered by active health measures. If a hormonal problem is going to occur, then it will, and there's little that can be done. Is this true?

No. There are many measures people can take to maintain the health and balance of the hormonal system. Some are similar to health measures for other body systems, including regular exercise for physical fitness, and an adequate diet with a range of **nutrients**. Indeed an unhealthy diet, especially being obese (overweight), is linked to several hormonal problems. These include certain forms of **diabetes mellitus**, and **thyroid** disorders. Lack of the **mineral** substance iodine in the diet can lead to one type of the enlarged thyroid known as goitre, as the thyroid **gland** becomes overactive.

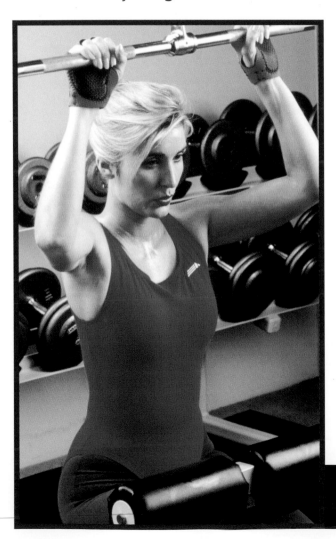

Physical damage

Physical injury or damage may disrupt the delicate function of hormone glands. For example, a constriction around the neck may rupture the thyroid, with widespread effects on body **metabolism**.

A head injury is often serious enough, with possible effects on the brain. It can also damage the dual controllers of the hormonal system, the **hypothalamus** and **pituitary**, with extensive and long-term effects throughout the body. One form of diabetes, known as diabetes insipidus, is most commonly caused by head injuries. This is another reason for using protective clothing and equipment, like wearing a helmet when cycling or playing extreme sports.

Suitable exercise benefits all body systems, including the hormonal system.

Chemical damage

Excessive alcohol harms many body parts, especially the liver and brain. It can also disrupt the general functions of the hormonal system. Likewise nicotine in tobacco, and many illegal drugs, also affect hormone function. This may be unclear at first, because it can take weeks or months to develop. Drug abuse has been linked especially to problems of the thyroid and adrenal glands.

Medical causes

In very rare cases, a hormonal problem is linked to medical treatment for another condition. Delicate surgery, certain medicinal drugs, or **radiotherapy** –

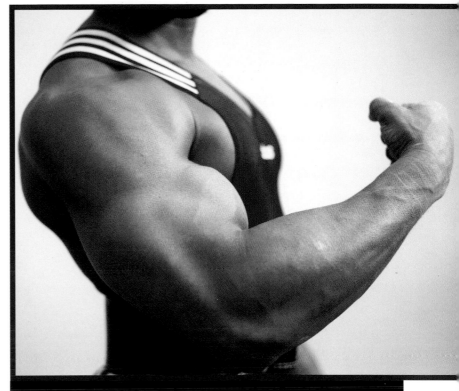

Anabolic steroids used by some bodybuilders to enhance muscle growth and physical performance, can have serious effects on long-term health.

the use of radiation or rays, for example, to kill off growths or **tumours** – may carry the risk of hormonal side effects. One example is unavoidable damage to an **endocrine** gland. Such risks are discussed with the patient before treatment. Should a hormonal condition result, this is usually easily treatable, and less serious than the original condition.

Steroid abuse

Some sports people resort to the use of drugs such as **steroids**. The sports involved may be those where muscle bulk is important, such as sprinting, weightlifting and bodybuilding. Many steroid drugs are artificial copies of the body's natural steroid hormones. One of their effects at normal levels is on muscles, but when steroids are boosted artificially, they can lead to numerous problems in other body parts. These include mood swings, digestive complaints, a deeper voice, excessive body hair and long-term problems of the **reproductive system** – even the inability to have children.

MAIN HORMONAL GLAND

The **pituitary** is in the middle of the head. It is under the base of the brain, in the centre towards the front, and just above the rear of the roof of the mouth. It is only the size of a large baked bean. The hormones and other substances it makes each day, if dried out into powder form, would be about the size of one tiny grain of salt. Yet the pituitary is the hormonal 'master **gland**'. It has great effects on many other parts of the hormonal system.

Hormones control hormones

The pituitary makes and/or releases more than ten hormones and other hormone-like substances. In addition, it is joined by a short stalk to the brain just above, and it is the main link between the two control

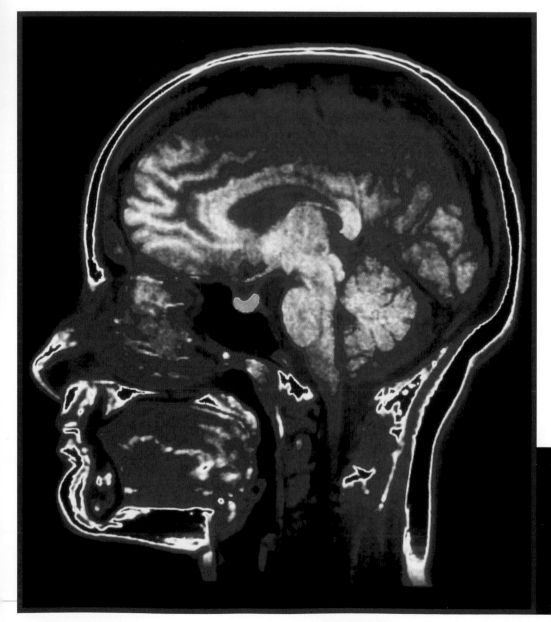

In this computerized scan through the head and brain, the pituitary is shown in green.

and coordination systems of hormones and nerves. Also, many pituitary hormones have targets that are other **endocrine** glands. So the pituitary is vital for the coordinated working of the whole hormonal system.

Two glands in one

The pituitary is not really a single gland, but two glands, one behind the other. The front one is known as the anterior pituitary. The rear one is the posterior pituitary. These two parts of the pituitary work in different ways, make different hormones and have different types of links with the **hypothalamus**.

The hypothalamus, just above the pituitary, is part of the brain that is important in very basic, life-maintaining functions. It helps to control body temperature. It is responsible for feelings of hunger and thirst, and so ensures that the body takes in enough food and water. It regulates sleep and waking. It is also important in strong emotions such as fear, anger, rage and great pleasure.

The pituitary may be the 'master gland' of the hormonal system, but in turn it is largely under control of the hypothalamus just above it. The links between the two, and the ways that the hypothalamus affects the pituitary, which then regulates many endocrine glands, are shown on the next few pages.

Position of the pituitary

The pituitary sits in a small, bowl-like notch or depression in one of the skull bones, the sphenoid. It is well protected from physical damage by this bone to its sides and below. Above, the pituitary is covered by a tough **membrane** that wraps around the stalk connecting it to the brain. Just above the membrane are main nerves from the eyes to the brain. If the pituitary enlarges, as may happen with a pituitary **tumour**, it may press on these nerves and cause problems with vision.

'Slime gland'

In the language of Latin, the name 'pituitary' means 'mucus' or 'slime'. The pituitary received this name because it was thought that the brain made slimy mucus, and the pituitary passed this on to the inside of the nose.

The anterior **pituitary** makes up about three-quarters of the bulk of the pituitary **gland**. Its microscopic cells make at least seven important hormones. One of the most important is growth hormone, which controls the body's overall physical growth, as you develop from a baby, through childhood and adolescence, into an adult.

Two supplies of blood

The anterior pituitary's hormones, listed below, pass into the normal blood supply flowing through it. The anterior pituitary has another, second blood supply, direct from the **hypothalamus** just above it. This blood flows from the hypothalamus along tiny tubes into the anterior pituitary.

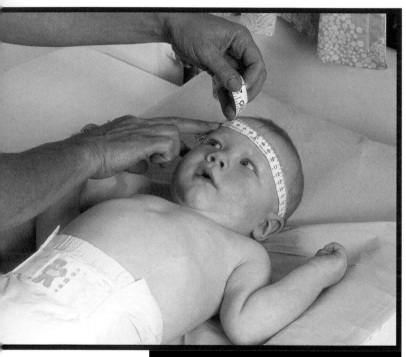

Check-ups detect if a baby is growing slowly due to lack of growth hormone.

Three-hormone system

The anterior pituitary makes its own hormones, and releases them into the general bloodstream. It does so largely under the control of other hormones, made in the hypothalamus. For each hormone of the anterior pituitary, there is a 'releasing' hormone from the hypothalamus. In turn, many anterior pituitary hormones exert their effects on other **endocrine** glands around the body. So there is a three-hormone control system: Releasing hormone (hypothalamus) > Control hormone (anterior pituitary) > Target hormone (endocrine gland).

Growth hormone (GH)

Growth hormone stimulates cells to multiply and make more **proteins**, which are the body's 'building block' substances. Different parts, such as bones and muscles, grow at their own natural rates as the body increases in size and changes in proportions, from baby to adult. Production of growth hormone is controlled by two hormones from the hypothalamus, GHRH (growth hormone releasing hormone) and GHIH (growth hormone inhibiting hormone).

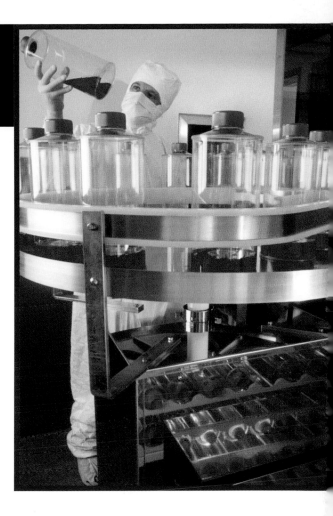

Some human hormones, such as growth hormone, can be made in the laboratory by microbes which have had their genes altered (**genetically engineered**).

Affecting other glands

Thyroid-stimulating hormone (TSH) regulates the gland called the thyroid, in the neck. It is regulated by TRH (thyrotropin-releasing hormone) from the hypothalamus. Adreno-corticotrophic hormone's (ACTH) targets are the adrenal glands, which are involved in the body's reactions to **stress**, pain and similar situations. Its control hormone from the hypothalamus is CRH (corticotropin-releasing hormone). These two examples show how important the anterior pituitary is to the **endocrine system** as a whole.

Luteinizing hormone (LH) and follicle-stimulating hormone (FSH) are mainly involved with the **reproductive system**. They are released during the teenage years, and stimulate the changes in the body that we call **puberty**. Prolactin is also associated with the reproductive system – it enables mothers to produce milk to feed their newborn babies.

Melanocyte-stimulating hormone (MSH)

Little is know about MSH. It seems to affect the cells called melanocytes in the skin. These make the dark substance melanin that gives skin its colour.

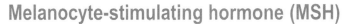

Monitoring growth

Many factors affect how fast and tall a child grows. They include the parents' height, ethnic group, diet and living conditions. In rare cases the anterior pituitary makes too little, or too much, growth hormone and this affects growth. However, most growth hormone problems are detected early, by measurements at regular health checks, and then analysis of blood samples for levels of the hormone. In most cases, the problem can be treated to restore normal growth. This is one reason why it is so important for babies and children to attend their regular medical check-ups.

The posterior **pituitary** makes up only one-quarter of the whole pituitary **gland**. It releases two hormones; antidiuretic hormone (ADH) and oxytocin, but it does not actually make them. The hormones are produced in the part of the brain just above, the **hypothalamus**. The hormones are released into the blood passing through the posterior pituitary.

Oxytocin

This hormone, like prolactin released from the anterior pituitary, is mainly involved in childbirth, and in the mother's release of milk for her new baby.

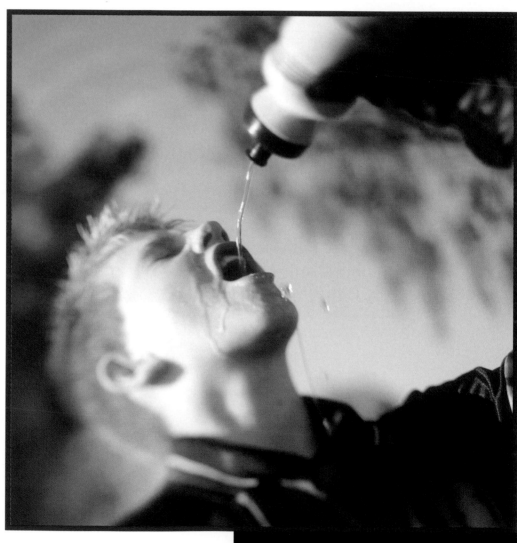

ADH controls the body's water balance. Feelings of thirst come about when water levels fall.

Antidiuretic hormone (ADH)

Antidiuretic hormone is involved in the body's overall water balance. The amount of water in the body must be delicately controlled within narrow limits, so that all parts can work efficiently, without being too dry or becoming flooded. If the body has too much or too little water, its cells can be damaged. Every time you feel thirsty, this is a result of water shortage in the body, and it involves the hormone ADH.

The body takes in water mainly by drinking. It gets rid of excess water mainly through the **kidneys**, as urine. The kidneys are ADH's main targets. Sensor cells in the hypothalamus detect a shortage of water in the body. They send nerve signals to the ADH-making cells nearby, which in turn send ADH and nerve signals down their fibres, to the fibre ends in the posterior pituitary. The fibre ends then release ADH into the bloodstream.

Conserving water

A diuretic substance increases urine production, while an antidiuretic has the opposite effect. Antidiuretic hormone affects the kidneys by making them produce less urine, and by making this urine more concentrated, that is, containing less water and more body wastes. These actions, along with taking in more water by drinking, raise the amount of water in the body and restore the water balance. Throughout a typical day, as you carry out exercise and sweat, then rest, and then eat and drink, levels of ADH rise and fall to maintain the body's vital water balance.

ADH and drugs

Certain drugs can affect ADH. In some cases, this can pose risks to the body's kidneys, and to its entire water and fluid balance. Nicotine (in tobacco) and **barbiturates** increase the release of ADH. This makes the kidneys produce less urine that is also more concentrated. The amount of water in the body rises, which can raise blood pressure, with possibly harmful effects as the heart works harder to pump blood around the body. Alcohol lowers the release of ADH. It makes the body produce more and less concentrated urine. Drinking alcohol makes people urinate more. However, as the body's water level falls, and thirst grows, taking another alcoholic drink only worsens the situation.

PITUITARY PROBLEMS

A problem in the **pituitary gland** can have widespread effects on the body. This is partly because the pituitary produces many hormones and these in turn control other hormonal glands. In particular, regular check-ups on growing babies and children are very important.

Growth hormone disorders

Too little or too much growth hormone can affect a baby or child. Such cases are rare. They may occur from birth or during childhood. Sometimes the cause is unknown. In other cases it is due to a growth or **tumour** in the pituitary or to physical damage, perhaps caused by a head injury.

Lack of growth hormone means a child increases in size slowly and is small for its age. Treatment is by regular injections of growth hormone. This used to be obtained from dead bodies, but is now made in **biotechnology** centres, using **genetically engineered** microbes.

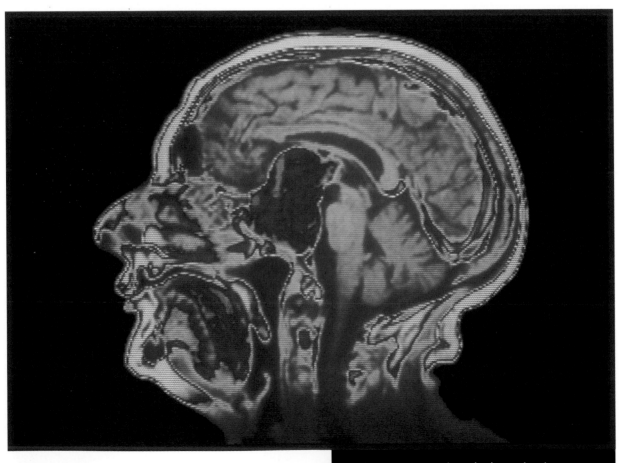

The pituitary, just below the lower front of the brain, can enlarge due to a tumour (centre, in pink).

The opposite problem is too much growth hormone leading to extra-fast growth. This can also be detected at an early stage and treated, in this case by tablets that lower the levels of growth hormone produced by the body.

Acromegaly

In rare cases excess growth hormone occurs in an adult, after normal growth has stopped. It causes acromegaly, which does not involve an increase in height, but renewed growth of the body's peripheral parts or extremities. These include the hands, feet, jaw, brow, nose and ears. The skin may become thicker and coarser, with tingling in the arms and legs. Treatment usually involves tablets to lower the hormone level, and perhaps surgery to correct the cause, such as a pituitary tumour.

Pituitary growths

Various types of growths or tumours can appear in the pituitary gland, nearly always in the anterior part. In many cases the reasons are not known. One type is an adenoma, an overgrowth of the normal hormone-making cells. This produces extra amounts of the hormones normally made in the pituitary gland, which can cause various problems. Raised levels of prolactin, for example, may lead to breast milk being made when not feeding a baby. This is called galactorrhea.

An enlarged pituitary growth may press on the adjacent nerves from the eyes to the brain, causing disturbed vision and headaches. Treatments for a pituitary tumour depend on the size and position of the growth, and its effects on the body. They include surgery, **radiotherapy**, or cryotherapy where the tumour is frozen by extreme cold from a narrow probe.

Diabetes insipidus

In this form of diabetes, the posterior pituitary does not produce enough antidiuretic hormone, ADH, so the **kidneys** do not conserve water effectively. The result is that the person produces a lot of very weak or dilute urine, and also feels continually thirsty and has to drink large amounts to replace the lost water. Causes include a head injury that damages the pituitary, or a tumour there. Treatment may be tablets to make the kidneys conserve water directly, or an artificial form of the hormone ADH that takes the place of the missing natural ADH. **Diabetes mellitus** is a different and more common condition, see page 30.

If a bow tie could be worn around the neck, but just under the skin instead of above it, this would show the size, shape and position of the **thyroid**. The **gland** has two **lobes**, one either side of the windpipe, with a narrower connecting portion, the isthmus. The thyroid makes the hormones thyroxine and tri-iodothyronine. It also produces calcitonin, the effects of which are described on page 22.

What do thyroid hormones do?

Thyroxine makes up about nine-tenths of the thyroid's total hormone output. Its targets are almost all body cells. This hormone makes cells work faster and carry out their chemical processes, known as **metabolism**, more rapidly. The cells use more oxygen and energy. They also generate more heat, and this warms the body. Cells in the brain, spleen and male sex glands are among the few which are hardly affected by thyroid hormones.

Also, during the first 15–20 years of life, thyroxine and other thyroid hormones act with growth hormone from the **pituitary**, to control growth and development. They are especially important for healthy development of bones and nerves. If thyroid hormones are lacking in a baby or child, physical growth and mental development are very slow, resulting in the medical condition known as cretinism.

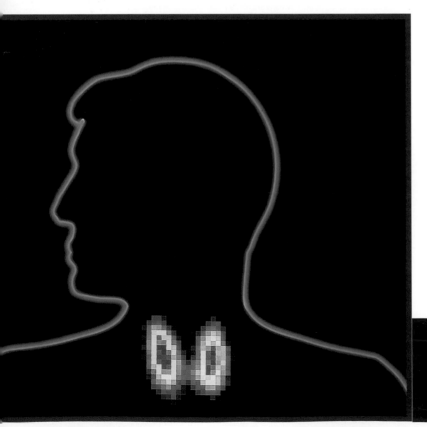

Too much thyroxine increases metabolic rate, while too little does the opposite. Thyroid-stimulating hormone (TSH) from the pituitary controls the release of thyroid hormones. This gives a balance between 'fast' and 'slow', so that the body functions normally and maintains a constant temperature. Thyroid problems can cause the body to 'go slow' and cool down, or even go fast and almost 'burn up'.

The thyroid gland is about the same size and shape as a 'bow tie' just under the skin of the neck.

Need for iodine

Thyroxine contains the **mineral** iodine. A **molecule** of thyroxine has four iodine **atoms**. (This gives rise to its shortened name, T4.) The regular supply of iodine, needed to make the hormone, comes from food. If iodine is lacking in the diet, this can cause a type of goitre.

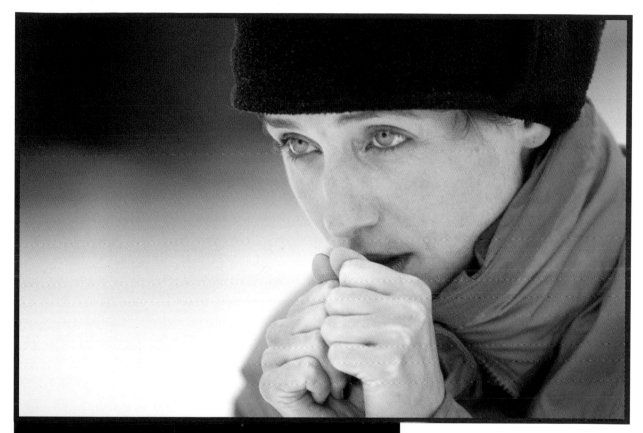

Our bodies have some natural defences against the cold. These include shivering and the release of hormones to generate heat.

Goitre

A goitre is an enlarged or swollen thyroid gland, seen as a lump in the front of the neck. There are several types and causes of goitre. In a simple or non-toxic goitre, the mineral iodine is lacking in food, so the thyroid cannot make enough thyroxine. The pituitary detects this via the feedback loop and releases more TSH, trying to make the thyroid grow and produce more hormones. Treatment is more iodine in the diet, found especially in fish, fish products and sea salt. Most types of table salt have small amounts of added iodine to prevent simple goitre.

PARATHYROIDS

There are four parathyroid **glands**, each about the size of a shirt button, on the rear of the **thyroid** gland. They make PTH, parathormone, which regulates the levels of two **minerals** in the body, calcium and phosphate.

The body uses calcium and phosphate to build and maintain strong bones and teeth. Calcium is also important in blood clotting, to seal wounds. A specific balance of calcium and phosphate is needed for healthy nerves, so they can pass their signals around the body, and control the heart and muscles.

The parathyroid glands are especially important during childhood and adolescence, as the bones enlarge and mature. However they are at risk from general 'hormonal collapse' caused by certain illegal drugs, or from physical injury to the neck region.

How parathormone works

Parathormone works with calcitonin from the thyroid gland, as described on page 20. These two hormones have opposing effects. Calcitonin lowers the level of calcium in the blood, while PTH raises it. If the blood level of calcium drops too low, the parathyroids release more PTH while the thyroid releases less calcitonin. PTH acts in several ways:

- it allows tiny amounts of bone to break down, and release their calcium into the bloodstream. (In a healthy body this does not cause problems, since bones have calcium in reserve.)
- it encourages more calcium and phosphate to be taken in from digested food. **Vitamin** D is needed for this process, another reason for a healthy diet with plenty of vitamins.
- it makes the **kidneys** conserve calcium within the body, rather than losing it in urine.

Actions of calcitonin

In general, calcitonin opposes the effects of PTH on the bones. However it is not an exact opposite. It tends to act over the short-term of hours and days, while PTH controls calcium over the long-term of months and years. Even so, working as a dual 'push-pull' system, PTH and calcitonin balance calcium levels within narrow limits, for good health. Several other sets of hormones have this 'push-pull' relationship.

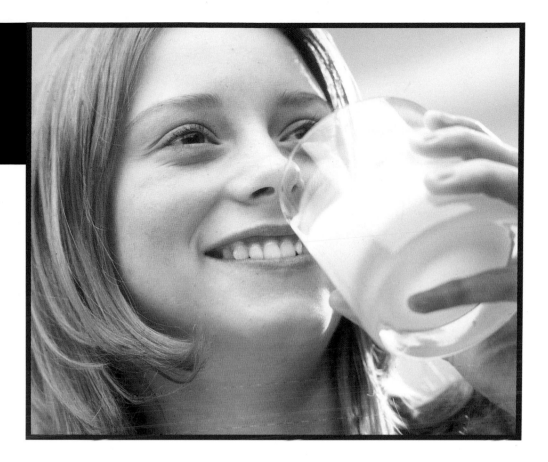

Calcium taken in from milk is regulated by parathyroid hormones.

Too much PTH

The parathyroids sometimes make too much PTH, which raises the body's calcium to abnormal levels. The most common cause of this condition (hyperparathyroidism) is a growth in one or more of the parathyroid glands. As calcium is taken from the bones to maintain its high level in the blood, the bones become weak and brittle. Other symptoms include indigestion and depression. Also, too much calcium passing from the blood, through the kidneys into the urine, may lead to kidney stones. Treatments include vitamin and mineral supplements, or surgery to remove the growth, or to remove up to three of the whole glands.

Underactive parathyroids

If the parathyroids are underactive (hypoparathyroidism), too little PTH drives calcium levels down. This produces painful cramps or spasms of the muscles, because faulty nerve signals make them contract abnormally. There may also be tingling and numbness, eye cataracts, dry skin and hair thinning. A child may even suffer headaches, convulsions and slow mental development. The major treatment is tablets of vitamin D to boost calcium levels towards normal.

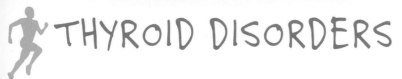

In a car, pressing the accelerator increases speed, while releasing it lets the car slow down. The **thyroid** is the body's 'accelerator'. Too much of its two main hormones makes cells work faster, and the whole body 'speeds up' – physically, chemically and mentally.

Too fast

Overactive thyroid **gland** can be known as hyperthyroidism, thyrotoxicosis, toxic goitre, Graves' disease, Basedow's disease or Plummer's disease, partly depending on the cause. In most cases, the problem is in the thyroid's control system. The thyroid is normally regulated by thyroid-stimulating hormone (TSH) from the **pituitary**, but an abnormal pituitary may produce too much TSH. This causes the thyroid to make too many hormones. A growth, nodule or **tumour** in the thyroid may also make excessive hormones.

The speeded-up body

Overactive thyroid affects about one person in 3,000; more than four out of five cases are in adult women. The extra thyroid hormones speed up body systems. The affected person is nervous, anxious, trembling, tired yet unable to sleep, rarely feels cold, and has a racing heart, weak muscles, digestive upsets and scanty menstrual periods. Appetite goes up, yet energy use is so great, body weight goes down. The eyes may be irritated and red, with double vision, and they appear to protrude or 'stare' – a condition called exophthalmos.

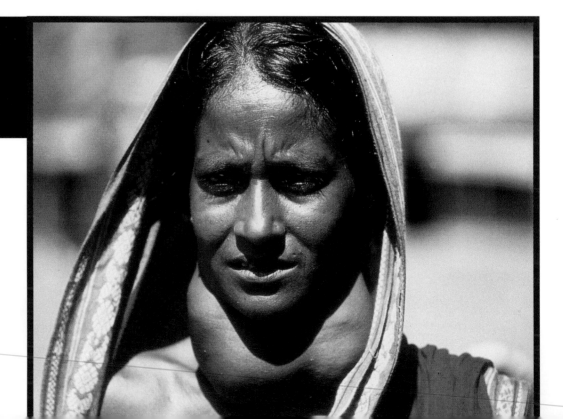

A goitre is a lump in the neck, which is an enlarged thyroid gland.

Too slow

Underactive thyroid gland is known as hypothyroidism. Causes include a fault with the thyroid's control system, such as too little TSH from the pituitary, or lack of the **mineral** iodine in food. The effects in a baby or child have already been described. In a rare form, Hashimoto's disease, the thyroid is gradually destroyed by substances called **antibodies**.

Lack of thyroid hormones makes the body slow down. The affected person is tired and listless, cannot concentrate, feels the cold and gains weight, with general pains, slowed heartbeat, constipation and heavier menstrual periods. A mucus-like substance collects in the skin and other body parts. It makes the face and skin look puffy, which is known as myxoedema.

Treatments

Thyroid problems have various treatments, depending on the cause. They include surgery and **radiotherapy** to remove growths from the thyroid. Dietary supplements, and various drugs, such as tablets of artificial thyroxine, can restore the balance of the body's hormones. In the great majority of cases, treatment is very effective.

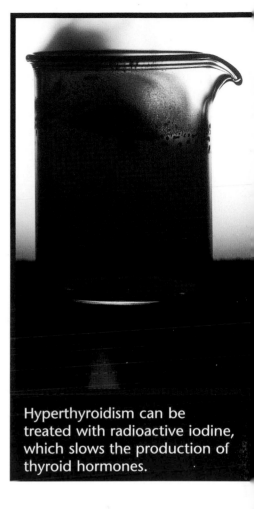

Hyperthyroidism can be treated with radioactive iodine, which slows the production of thyroid hormones.

Feel cold, get warm

The body normally maintains a temperature of about 37°Celsius. If body temperature falls below this, internal temperature sensors in the brain detect it, causing a three-linked hormone reaction:
- the sensors tell the **hypothalamus** to release more TRH
- TRH tells the pituitary to release more TSH
- TSH tells the thyroid to release more thyroxine.
The thyroid hormones tell cells to speed up and produce more heat, restoring body temperature to normal.

In some conditions your body might be unable to regulate its temperature, because of extreme cold, or lack of food to produce more heat for the body. If body temperature falls below 35°C, **hypothermia** can set in. If the body temperature continues to fall, the patient may eventually lose consciousness and die.

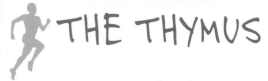

The thymus is an unusual multi-purpose **gland** in the front of the chest, just behind the upper breastbone, in front of the heart and lungs. It is soft and pinkish-grey, and has two main parts or **lobes**, joined by strong connective tissue.

In proportion to the whole body, the thymus is biggest in a newborn baby (about the size of the baby's clenched fist). It enlarges to about twice this size by early adolescence, although the rest of the body grows much more. The thymus is also most active during childhood and early adolescence. As the body becomes fully-grown and mature, the thymus begins to shrink. It continues to get smaller with age, but never quite disappears. Whether it becomes inactive in old age is a matter of debate. It can be removed during adulthood with no apparent side effects.

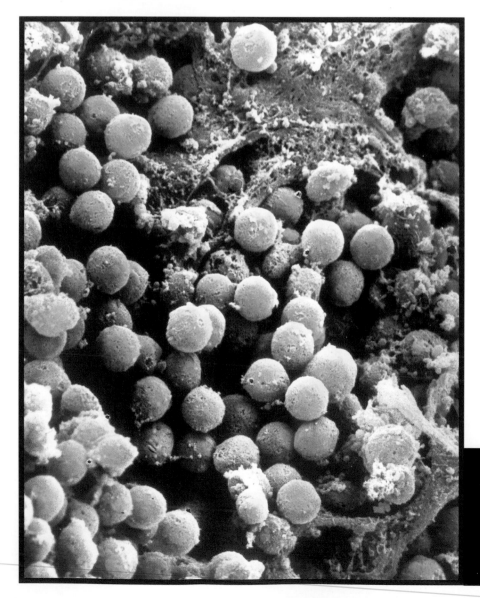

These ball shapes are disease-fighting T-lymphocyte blood cells in the thymus.

Many roles

The thymus has several roles. It works as a lymph gland of the **lymphatic system**, which involves the slowly circulating fluid, lymph, formed from tissue fluid that collects between cells and tissues. The spleen and tonsils are also parts of the lymphatic system, which filters waste material out of the lymph before returning it to the circulating blood. Another major role for the thymus is in the **immune system,** which protects the body from infection by germs and other diseases.

Thymus hormones

The thymus makes hormones and hormone-like substances known as factors, which have effects on both the immune and **reproductive systems**. There are at least ten of these hormones and factors, most importantly thymosin.

One of the thymus's hormonal roles is to process cells from the **bone marrow** into specialized cells of the immune system, able to fight infection. They become types of white blood cells known as T-lymphocytes ('T' for 'thymus-derived' or 'thymus-dependent'). The thymus manufactures hormones for this purpose, which assist the cells to become specialized, and which also maintain these cells in various parts of the body, so they are always ready to battle against disease.

Germ warfare

Thymus hormones also take part in another process of the immune system. They help certain other white blood cells, known as B-lymphocytes, to become specialized into **plasma** cells. The plasma cells then produce substances called **antibodies**, which stick on to invading germs and damage or disable them. If the thymus has not fully developed in a baby, or is removed in early life, the immune system is unable to develop completely.

The thymus and the reproductive system

Thymus hormones and factors have effects on the master gland of the hormonal system, the **pituitary**. In particular, they affect the production of reproductive and sex hormones such as luteinizing hormone (LH) and follicle-stimulating hormone (FSH) from the pituitary. However their exact role in the reproductive system, and whether these thymus hormones help the body to become sexually mature during **puberty,** is not clear.

HORMONES OF THE PANCREAS

Cars run on petrol. The body's 'petrol' – its main energy-giving fuel – is the sugar **glucose**. Its levels in the blood and cells, and its use by various body parts, is controlled by hormones from the **pancreas**. This large, soft, wedge-shaped **gland** is in the upper left abdomen, behind the stomach. It looks like one gland, but it works as two. It has vital roles in both the hormonal and **digestive systems**. For digestion, it makes powerful chemicals known as **enzymes**. These pass along a tube, the pancreatic duct, into the intestine and break down food.

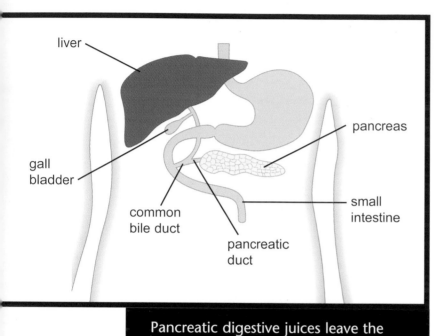

Pancreatic digestive juices leave the pancreas via a duct. Its hormones leave in the blood supply.

Blood sugar

The pancreas makes the hormones **insulin** and glucagon. Along with another hormone from the adrenal glands, insulin and glucagon control the level of blood glucose. Cells take in glucose from the blood, and break it apart to release the energy it contains. This energy powers their many chemical processes. The level or concentration of glucose in the blood is regulated within narrow limits by the two pancreatic hormones. Too much or too little glucose, in blood and body tissues, can cause serious health problems as described over the page.

Effects of insulin

1 Insulin makes many body cells take in glucose from the blood, to use or store.
2 It encourages the liver to take in **molecules** of glucose, and join them together to produce much bigger molecules of another substance, glycogen (a form of starch). This acts as a longer-term store of energy.
3 It encourages cells in fatty or adipose tissue to take in glucose, and convert it into fat.
4 It allows cells to take in substances called **amino acids** more easily, and use them to build **proteins**, which form the structural framework of many body parts.

Overall, the first three effects of insulin make the level of blood glucose fall, the second and third increase the body's longer-term energy stores, and the last two build new body tissues.

The effects of glucagon

Glucagon encourages cells in the liver to break apart their glycogen into separate glucose molecules, which pass into the blood. Glucagon also encourages other substances, such as amino acids and lactic acids, to be changed into glucose. (The hormone cortisol from the adrenal glands also does this, as shown later.) Both these actions raise the level of glucose in the blood.

Working together

By working together, insulin and glucagon regulate the level of blood glucose. If the level falls too low, the pancreas releases more glucagon and less insulin. If the glucose level becomes too high, the reverse occurs. This happens almost every minute of every day.

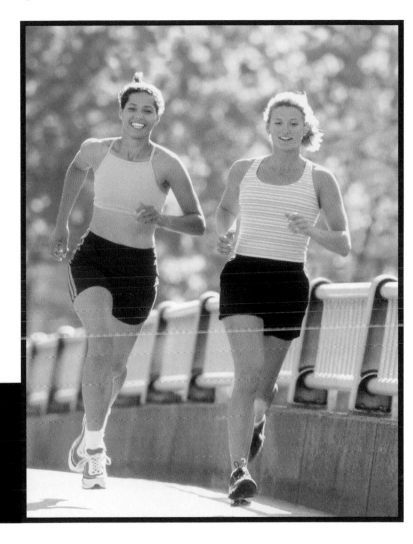

Exercise and sports 'burn' glucose, which releases its energy for muscles.

Meals and sports

The body's need for a quickly available energy source, blood glucose, varies hugely throughout the day. When you are very active, exercising or playing sport, your muscles use glucose fast. So the pancreas releases glucagon, which stimulates the liver to convert its store of glycogen into glucose. This continually tops up your level of blood glucose. When you eat a large meal, or a sugary chocolate bar, the glucose digested from it floods into the blood. The pancreas releases plenty of insulin to lower the glucose level, by converting it into glycogen in the liver.

PROBLEMS OF THE PANCREAS

The **pancreas**, like other body parts, can be affected by various disorders, such as inflammation, infections and growths. These may disrupt both its digestive and hormonal roles. The major hormone-related condition affecting the pancreas is **diabetes mellitus**, sometimes called sugar diabetes. (A different condition, diabetes insipidus, is described on page 19.)

Lack of insulin

In diabetes mellitus, the pancreas produces too little or no **insulin**. As a result, cells cannot take up enough high-energy **glucose**, and the blood glucose level rises too high.

More urine, more thirst

Symptoms of diabetes include large volumes of urine, and great thirst to replace the water lost. Inability to use glucose for energy causes tiredness and weakness. Associated symptoms are muscle cramps, tingling hands and feet, blurred vision, and perhaps weight loss. Menstrual periods may also be disturbed. There is general lowered resistance to infection, especially in the urinary tract, where sugar in the urine encourages germs to breed. The brain also needs a supply of glucose – if this doesn't happen it can, in extreme cases, lead to brain damage.

Different forms

There are two different forms of diabetes mellitus. Type 1, or insulin-dependent diabetes, normally develops before the age of 20. The body cannot produce insulin because the insulin-producing cells of the pancreas have been destroyed by the body's own **immune system**. Type 2 can appear in later life, because insulin production slows down or the body's cells no longer respond to the insulin.

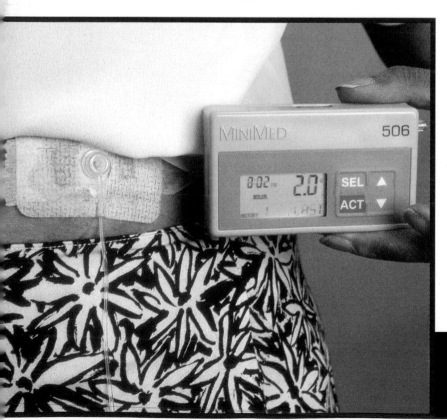

Electronic devices measure blood glucose level and inject insulin accordingly.

Although there is probably a **genetic** reason why Type 2 develops, it is closely linked to poor diet, obesity, lack of exercise and smoking. Type 2 is the more common form of diabetes mellitus.

Careful monitoring

A person with diabetes needs to keep a close control on what he or she eats and drinks. Care is needed before and after physical activities such as sports, which use energy. However, the condition is not necessarily a problem – many people with diabetes have risen to the top of their sport. It is important for diabetics to monitor their blood sugar level carefully, and take steps to keep the level constant.

Type 1 diabetics need to inject themselves with insulin to replace the body's missing supply. The insulin used to be obtained from animals such as cows and sheep. It can now be made in **biotechnology** centres, using **genetically engineered** microbes. This needs to be matched by eating foods that raise the blood sugar level slowly. Examples include foods like potatoes, pulses and cereals, which are high in **carbohydrates**.

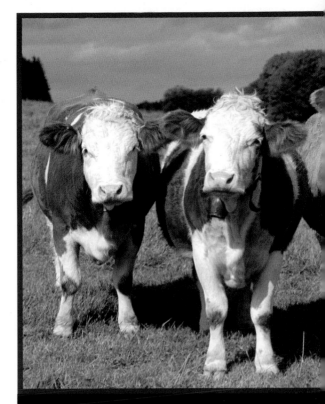

Before scientists discovered how to produce insulin, Type 1 diabetics relied on insulin from animals such as cows.

Type 2 diabetes is managed by avoiding sugary foods, and replacing them with foods that raise blood sugar level slowly. Sufferers also need to cut down alcohol intake, stop smoking and take more exercise.

Hypoglycaemia

Hypoglycaemia is the result of very low blood glucose. Causes include disrupted treatment of diabetes, another hormonal problem such as underactive **pituitary**, or pancreatic disease. The person becomes sweaty, dizzy, weak and confused, with slurred speech and blurred vision. He or she may turn aggressive or violent, and even collapse.

Hypoglycaemia is dangerous in itself. It may also be mistaken for the effects of alcohol or illegal drugs. This increases risks still further, since the sufferer may not receive the urgent treatment it requires – glucose tablets, sugary sweets or a glucose injection, to restore blood glucose level.

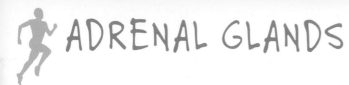

Some hormones work over the long-term, taking months or years to have their effects. Others act more quickly, in hours, minutes or even seconds. Several of the fastest-acting hormones are made by the adrenal **glands**. In particular, they help the body to cope with all kinds of **stress**, from mental worry and anxiety, to lack of food or water, an injury that needs repair, an infection or other disease, or a sudden emergency that demands immediate action.

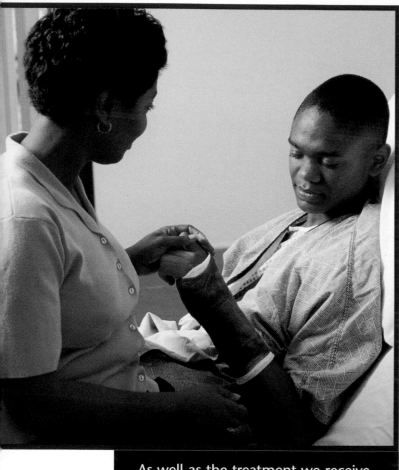

As well as the treatment we receive from doctors, hormones produced by the adrenal gland also help us to recover from an injury or infection.

The two **kidneys**, which filter waste from the blood to form the liquid urine, are also known as the renal glands. The adrenal glands are perched one on top of each kidney, and are also known as supra-renal glands. Each adrenal gland is shaped like a small, hollow bowl draped over the top of its kidney.

Two-in-one gland

Each adrenal is really two glands, one wrapped around the other. The outer part or layer is called the cortex, and makes up about nine-tenths of the bulk of the adrenal. The remainder is the inner, or central part, known as the medulla. Cortex and medulla have different types of cells, make different hormones with different chemical structures, and work in different ways on different targets. The cortex and medulla even originate from different body parts very early in life, in the **embryo** as it develops inside the womb.

Cortex

The adrenal cortex produces about five main hormones involved in the day-to-day running of the body; how it grows and develops, and how it reacts to low levels of **nutrients**, injury, illness, pain and other stressful but relatively common situations. These hormones are known as **steroids**, from their chemical structure. Other hormones control their amounts, and their targets include many parts of the body.

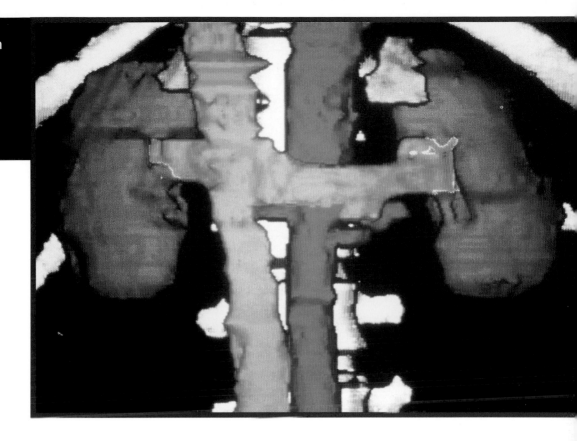

This body scan shows each adrenal gland (pink/purple) above its kidney (red).

Medulla

The adrenal medulla produces two major hormones, **adrenaline** and nor-adrenaline. Their amounts are controlled by the **nervous system**, rather than by other hormones. The targets of the adrenal medulla hormones are very specific, including the heart, blood vessels, muscles and **digestive system**. These hormones work with the nervous system to prepare the body for quick action in very demanding or extraordinary situations.

Both sets of hormones, from the cortex and medulla, are described in detail over the following pages.

The need for cholesterol

The substance cholesterol is often linked with the health of the heart and blood system. High levels of cholesterol in the blood can increase the risk of heart disease. Some cholesterol, however, is essential, since it is a raw material used in several ways by various body parts. The adrenal cortex needs cholesterol to make its steroid hormones. In fact the adrenal cortex has the highest levels, or concentrations, of cholesterol in the whole body. Cholesterol is present in fatty foods like dairy products.

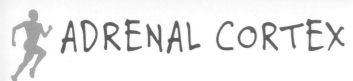

The adrenal cortex (outer layer) makes several important **steroid** hormones, known as corticoids. These have wide-ranging effects on the body in health, illness, growth and development. The main groups of these hormones are named from the main processes they control: glucocorticoids, mineralocorticoids and gonadocorticoids.

Sugar and fat

The chief glucocorticoids are cortisol (hydrocortisone) and corticosterone. Cortisol accounts for more than nine-tenths of the total. These two hormones help to control the level of the sugar **glucose** in the blood. Glucose is the body's readily available energy source. It is taken in and broken apart by cells, to release energy that drives their chemical processes.

Blood glucose is under the close control of several hormones, including **insulin** and glucagon from the **pancreas**. Cortisol causes the liver to make new supplies of glucose from the raw material of **proteins**, the main structural substances our bodies need for growth and repair. More cortisol causes blood glucose level to rise. In turn, the level of cortisol is controlled by adreno-corticotrophic hormone (ACTH) from the **pituitary gland**.

Cortisol has many other effects. It breaks down fatty substances so that they are also available as energy sources. It reduces the body's reactions to infection, disease or injury, by acting as an anti-inflammatory to reduce swelling, irritation, redness and pain. It also reduces allergic or immune reactions in a similar way. Cortisol also

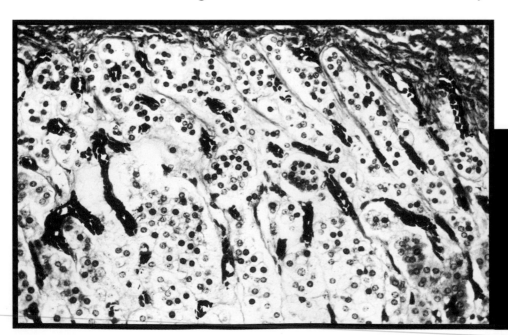

The adrenal cortex contains millions of hormone-making cells.

works with the **nervous system** and the hormones from the adrenal medulla, like **adrenaline**, to prepare the body for sudden action.

Minerals and blood pressure

Mineralocorticoids help to regulate **mineral nutrients** in the body. The main one, aldosterone, has the **kidneys** as its major targets. It makes the kidneys retain water and the mineral sodium in the body, while getting rid of potassium. It also reduces the loss of sodium in saliva, stomach juices and sweat. The balance of sodium and potassium gives body fluids the right amount of **acidity**. Also, conserving water and sodium increases the volume of the blood, and so keeps blood pressure at a healthy level. Aldosterone itself is controlled by a system that involves the **enzyme** renin, from the kidneys, and angiotensin, which circulates in the blood.

Sex organs

Gonadocorticoids include male sex hormones, called androgens, like testosterone, and female oestrogens. These affect the sex organs. They are particularly important for growth and sexual development during **puberty**.

Steroid drugs

There are many kinds of natural steroids in the body, including steroid hormones. There are also many kinds of steroid drugs available, for a wide variety of conditions.

Anti-inflammatory steroids have a similar action to cortisol. They reduce the swelling, redness, irritation and pain, during an inflammatory, immune or allergic reaction.

Anabolic steroids encourage the body to build up its tissue bulk, especially muscle.

Sex steroids have effects on the sex organs and also other parts of the body; some are anabolic. For example, the male sex hormones called androgens stimulate muscle growth, which is why men have relatively more muscle tissue for body size, compared to women.

Misuse or abuse of such drugs can have many adverse effects.

ADRENAL MEDULLA

Life has its ups and downs – a sometimes dull daily routine, but with the occasional worrying moment, fright or great excitement. Hormones play a vital part in helping the body to cope with the **stresses** of daily life. In particular, the inner part or medulla of the adrenal **gland** produces two main hormones. These are **adrenaline**, also known as epinephrine, and nor-adrenaline, also called nor-epinephrine. Normally adrenaline is produced in larger amounts than nor-adrenaline and has greater, more wide-ranging effects on the body.

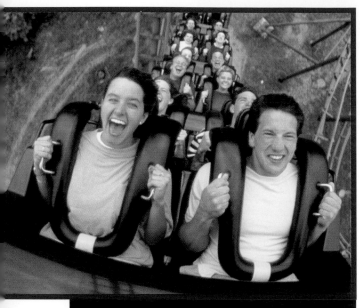

During a rollercoaster ride your body produces adrenaline hormones, causing your heart to race!

Nervous hormones

The microscopic cells that make up the adrenal medulla are similar to some of the cells that go to make up the **nervous system** in the earliest stages of an **embryo**. In some ways, the effects of adrenaline are more similar to those of nerves, than to the effects of other hormones. Adrenaline works very fast, in seconds. Its effects also fade away quickly, in minutes. Many of its targets are also controlled by nerves.

Effects of adrenaline

Adrenaline is sometimes called the 'fright, fight, flight' hormone, as described on page 38. Its actions are to prepare the body for sudden physical action. Some of its targets are:

- heart – the rate of beating (pulse-rate) increases, and extra blood is pumped with each beat
- blood vessels – the vessels to the heart muscle, and other muscles widen. This allows greater blood flow, but vessels to the skin narrow, turning skin pale.
- blood pressure – this rises as a result of the heart's faster, more powerful beats, and narrowed blood vessels in some body parts
- muscles – receive more blood, and are ready for action
- liver – increases breakdown of starch to provide **glucose** as a quickly available energy source for the blood and muscles
- lungs – the airways widen, and chest muscles work faster to increase breathing rate
- internal organs (stomach, intestines, sex organs) – blood flow reduces and muscles relax
- other hormones – decreases level of **insulin**, which allows blood glucose to rise and also provides other energy sources like fats, mainly for the muscles, brain and nerves.

Nor-adrenaline

The second hormone from the adrenal medulla, nor-adrenaline, has similar effects to adrenaline. However, these are generally less marked and less widespread. Nor-adrenaline widens the coronary arteries to the heart muscle, so that the heart can pump faster and more powerfully. It makes blood vessels in the skin and internal organs narrower. Nor-adrenaline also causes the **digestive system** to slow down, and it encourages fatty tissues to release their energy stores.

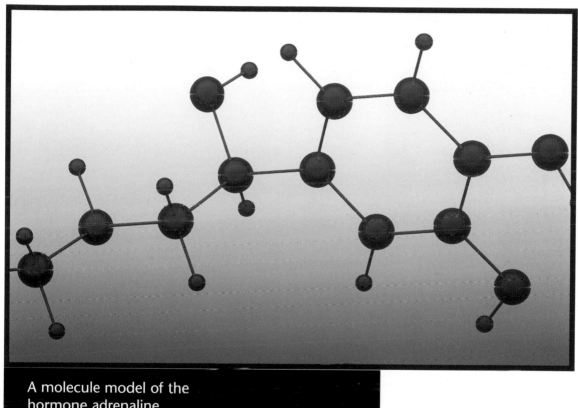

A molecule model of the hormone adrenaline.

Red alert!

The main aim of adrenaline is to make the body ready for sudden action, with heightened senses, increased alertness and fast responses. The heart, muscles and nervous system are speeded up. At the same time blood supply is reduced to the skin, stomach and other parts not important in physical activity, so that digestion and other internal systems slow down. The effects of adrenaline on the body mean that it can be used to treat anaphylactic shock. This is an extreme allergic reaction, for example to certain foods or drugs. It causes the blood pressure to drop alarmingly – airways narrow and skin becomes pale. Adrenaline can be injected to counteract these effects.

HORMONES AND STRESS

Imagine you are walking along the street one day. As you turn the corner you come face to face with – a lion! At once your heart pounds, your breathing quickens, your muscles tense and your body is ready for action. You have had a fright, and you are ready to stand and fight, or run away in flight. This is the 3F reaction – fright, fight or flight.

An unlikely event, perhaps, but **stress** is part of daily existence. The body adapts to cope with a certain amount of excitement and challenge. Otherwise life would be very dull and tedious. On the other hand, too much stress, or the wrong types of stress, can cause short-term illness and long-term health problems, both physical and mental.

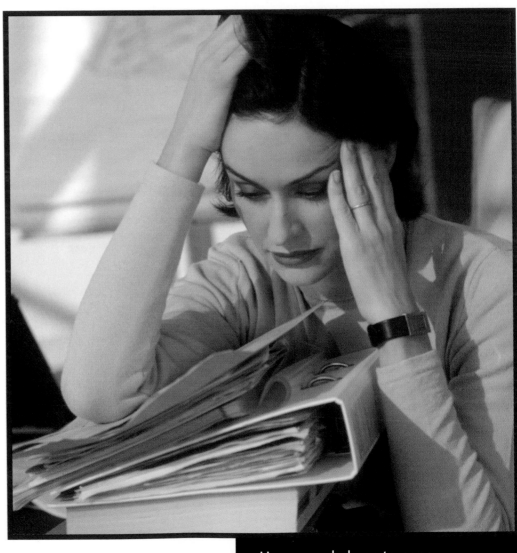

Hormones help us to cope with all kinds of stress – physical, mental (like exams) and emotional.

Hormones play a great part in the body's natural responses to stress. The adrenal **glands**, in particular, regulate internal processes that enable the body to get ready for action or cope with strain, physical and mental hardship, illness, pain and periods without food or drink.

The brain takes charge

The brain recognizes a stressful situation, as the conscious mind becomes aware of danger or problems. This sets off several chains of events. Most quickly, the brain sends signals through the **nervous system** to prepare the body for action. Heartbeat and breathing speed up to provide muscles with more oxygen and energy. Blood vessels to the muscles widen, while those to the inner organs and skin narrow, so the skin turns pale. Digestion is not essential and almost stops, so there is little saliva and the mouth feels dry. The skin also becomes sweaty, the eyes open wide, their pupils become wider too, and possibly hair stands on end.

Nerves and hormones

The brain also sends signals directly along nerves to the adrenal medulla, telling it to release **adrenaline** (see page 36). This hormone has many similar effects to the nerve responses listed above. It also helps to raise the level of blood **glucose** for available energy. The two systems, nervous and hormonal, support and reinforce each other.

Over the slightly longer-term, the brain also instructs the **pituitary** to release more adreno-corticotrophic hormone (ACTH), which tells the adrenal cortex to release more cortisol. This hormone allows some of the body's less essential structural **proteins** to be broken down. They are changed into glucose for energy, or used to build new tissues for the repair of wounds and injuries. Cortisol also encourages breakdown of stored fats, for use as an energy source.

Calming down

Some hormones are long-lived. After their release, they stay active in the blood for hours or days. Adrenaline is very short-lived. If the adrenal glands suddenly stopped releasing adrenaline, this hormone would be almost gone from the bloodstream within 3 minutes – inactivated and broken down by the liver. This is why, after a sudden fright that is a false alarm, the body calms down again quite quickly.

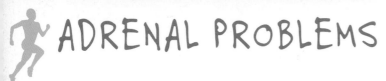

Like other hormone **glands**, the adrenal glands may be overactive and make too much of their hormones, or underactive and produce too little. Such cases are rare, especially in children. They are usually treated successfully with modern medicines and perhaps surgery. Some cases, however, are linked to **steroid** drugs (see panel).

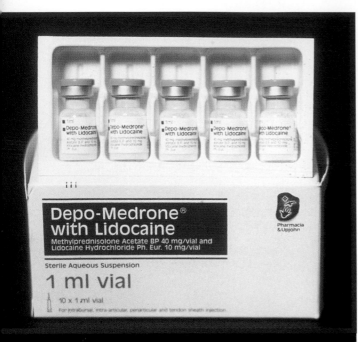

Many medications are based on natural corticoid hormones from the adrenal cortex. For example, depomedrone (shown here), which can be used to treat hay fever.

Cushing's syndrome

The adrenal cortex (outer layer) makes steroid hormones. If levels of these are too high, Cushing's syndrome can result. The body, shoulders, and noticeably the face, become rounder and fatter while their muscles shrink and weaken. The bones weaken too (osteoporosis), the skin develops streaks, spots and bruises, and there is general tiredness and depression. Other conditions may accompany these changes, such as **diabetes mellitus** or heart problems. In a woman the voice may deepen, with increased body hair and irregular periods.

Too much steroid

There are various causes of Cushing's syndrome. They include growths, or **tumours** in the adrenal glands that make excess hormones. A tumour in the **pituitary** may produce too much adreno-corticotrophic hormone (ACTH) which then over-stimulates the adrenal glands. In some cases the reason is use of **steroid** drugs, perhaps taken in large quantities to treat another serious disease, or used without medical supervision.

Underactive adrenal

If the adrenal cortex does not produce enough steroid hormones, the body can compensate to some extent. However, lack of cortisol may result in Addison's disease. The supply of energy-giving blood **glucose** is disrupted and the sufferer loses weight and appetite, feels tired and weak, and has digestive upsets. Also the skin darkens, almost like a suntan. Tablets of the hormone treat the condition, which is monitored to prevent another illness triggering acute adrenal failure.

High blood pressure

There are many causes of high blood pressure, and one occurs when the cortex of the adrenal produces too much of its hormone aldosterone. This may accompany another disease such as liver cirrhosis, or it can be due to a growth in one adrenal, when it is known as Conn's syndrome. Treating the other disease, or surgery to remove the growth, perhaps coupled with diuretic tablets, usually brings a great improvement.

Panic for no reason

In rare cases, a growth in the medulla of the adrenal gland makes too much **adrenaline**. Light exercise, exposure to cold, a slight emotional upset or even a small surprise can bring on the full adrenaline 'rush' of racing heart, panting, sweating and fear or panic. This condition is usually treated by an operation to remove the growth.

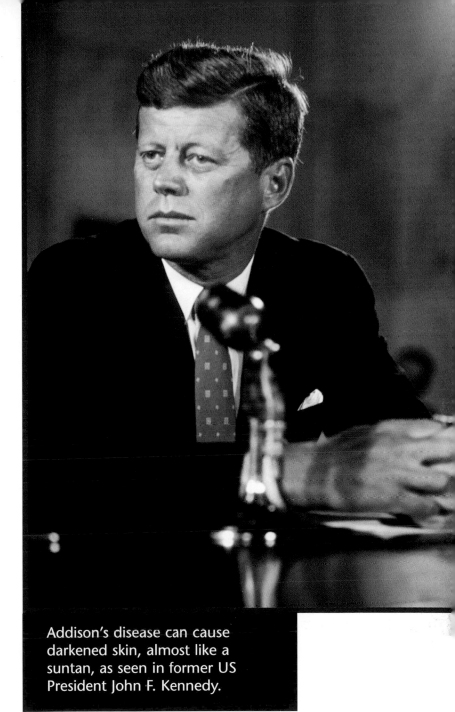

Addison's disease can cause darkened skin, almost like a suntan, as seen in former US President John F. Kennedy.

Steroid drug side effects

Modern steroid drugs, used under medical supervision, are very safe. Rarely they may produce a mild form of Cushing's syndrome. Usually a change of drug or treatment solves the problem. Patients are warned about suddenly stopping steroid drugs without medical approval. This could bring on acute adrenal failure, with serious weakness, confusion and collapse.

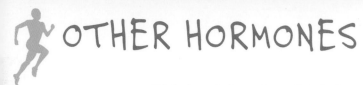

This book has described the body's main hormones or 'chemical messengers'. They help the body to grow, develop, become mature, regulate its internal conditions, maintain its health, fight illness and cope with **stress**. However, hormones are not automatic, anonymous substances that continue to work like clockwork, whatever happens. They are delicately balanced and responsive to change. Many aspects of lifestyle, such as diet, exercise and various drugs, affect them.

Other hormone makers

Most of the body parts shown in this book are **endocrine glands**. Other parts of the body, which have major tasks in other systems, make hormones too.

The heart makes atriopeptin (natriuretic factor, ANF). It affects the blood vessels, adrenal glands, **kidneys** and sensors in the brain. It is thought to help control blood pressure, and the balance of **minerals** and fluids in the body.

Digestive organs make several hormones. The stomach produces gastrin, which has itself as its target, producing acid to digest food. Secretin comes from the small intestine, and makes the **pancreas** release its digestive juices into the intestine. Cholecystokinin (CCK) from the same source has a similar action and also makes the gall bladder release the digestive juice called bile, into the intestine. The kidneys produce erythropoietin, which maintains or boosts the numbers of oxygen-carrying red cells in the blood. They also make renin, involved in control of blood pressure.

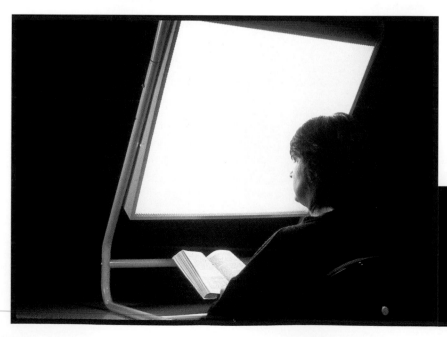

Phototherapy (light treatment) can help some people with seasonal affective disorder (SAD).

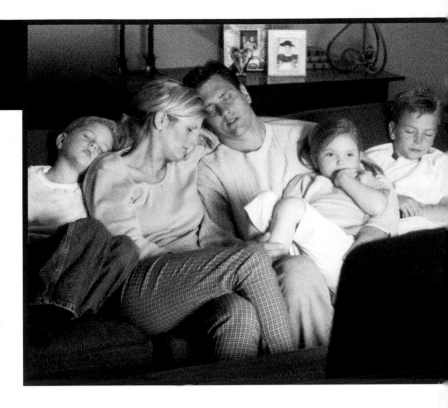

Late nights watching TV or using computers, disrupt many body systems.

The pineal

The pineal gland is deep inside the brain. It has links with the overall controllers of the hormonal system, the **hypothalamus** in the brain and the **pituitary** gland just below it. The pineal also links with the nerves that carry signals from the eyes through the brain, and especially with the brain's built-in 'body clock' or 'biological clock'.

Hormones and the body clock

The SCN 'body clock' coordinates a vast array of biorhythms. These are processes that vary in a regular and interlinked way, day and night. They include body temperature, hormone levels, urine formation, digestive activity, injury repair, **immune system** action, alertness, waking and sleep. The pineal gland works with the SCN, and is affected by nerve signals from the eyes, which bring information about levels of daylight and darkness. The pineal's main product is melatonin, known as the 'sleep hormone'. As darkness falls and melatonin levels rise in the evening, they bring on drowsiness and eventually sleep.

Rhythms and blues

The complex links between the SCN, the rest of the hypothalamus, the pineal gland's production of melatonin, and general body rhythms are easily disturbed. Very late nights, sudden early mornings, exercise at odd times, shift work, travelling across time zones, erratic mealtimes, and other changes to daily routine can all take their toll. Possible results include lack of energy, depression and sleeping problems. These are seen in jet lag, chronic fatigue syndrome (CFS), and seasonal affective disorder (SAD), which is believed to result from lack of daylight during long, dark winters.

We know much about the workings of the hormonal system. However, research into topics such as the effects of daylight, body rhythms and the role of the pineal gland, should bring exciting new information that could affect the way we carry out our daily lives.

This book has explained the different hormones and glands that control the functions of your body, why they are important and how they can be damaged by injury and illness. This page summarizes some of the problems that can affect hormones. It also gives you information about how each problem is treated.

Many health problems can also be avoided by good health behaviour. This is called prevention. Taking regular exercise and getting plenty of rest are important, as is eating a balanced diet. This is important in your teenage years, when your body is still developing. The table that follows tells you some of the ways you can prevent injury and illness.

Remember, if you think something is wrong with your body, you should always talk to a trained medical professional, like a doctor or a school nurse. Regular medical check-ups are an important part of maintaining a healthy body.

Illness or injury	Cause	Symptoms	Prevention	Treatment
Simple goitre	Mineral iodine is lacking in blood. The thyroid gland is unable to produce enough thyroxine. The pituitary releases more TSH to try and stimulate the thyroid.	The thyroid becomes overactive and swells, causing a lump to appear in the front of the neck.	Make sure your diet includes iodine. Fish, fish products and salt all contain iodine.	Treated by increasing iodine content of the diet.
Diabetes mellitus Type 1 – insulin dependent diabetes)	The body is unable to produce insulin, usually because of damage to the cells of the pancreas. This form of diabetes mellitus usually develops at a young age and is thought to have a genetic cause.	The body converts fats and proteins into energy, causing weight loss. These fats alter the pH of your blood – a sign of this being that breath smells of pear drops. Excretion of glucose uses water, which causes thirst and dehydration. Eventually, high blood pressure can damage blood vessels, leading to problems such as kidney failure.	This form of diabetes mellitus is not preventable, because it has genetic causes. The symptoms can be controlled (see treatment).	The condition can be managed by eating foods that raise blood sugar slowly, such as potatoes and cereals. This is combined with regular injections of insulin.

Illness or injury	Cause	Symptoms	Prevention	Treatment
Diabetes mellitus (Type 2 – non-insulin dependent diabetes)	Insulin production slows down or the body stops responding to the insulin circulating in the blood. Although this has some genetic causes it is affected by lifestyle factors such as poor diet, lack of exercise and smoking. Type 2 normally affects people over the age of 40.	As type 1 opposite.	Good health behaviour such as eating a balanced diet, taking plenty of exercise, not drinking too much alcohol and not smoking.	This form of diabetes mellitus is treated by a change of diet, to include more things like wholemeal bread and cereals, and by increasing exercise and cutting alcohol intake.
Addison's disease	Lack of cortisol being produced in the adrenal cortex, causing supply of blood glucose to be disrupted.	Feeling weak and lacking in energy, losing weight and appetite. Skin darkens.	Many adrenal problems are linked to the use of artificial steroids – this should be avoided.	Treated by tablets of the hormone. The disease needs careful monitoring.

Further reading

The Human Machine, The Controls: All about your brain, senses and nervous system, Sarah Angliss, Graham Rosewarne (Illustrator) (Belitha Press, 1999)
Human Physiology and Health, David Wright (Heinemann Educational, 2000)
Look at Your Body, Reproduction and Growing Up, Steve Parker (Franklin Watts, 1996)
Need to Know, Steroids, Sean Connolly (Heinemann Library, 2000)

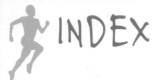